REVITALIZE

WITH

WATERCRESS

The ultimate guide to radiant well-being

Copyright © 2023 by Dr. Emmanuel Gold

All rights reserved. No part of this publication may be reproduced, distributed, or transmitted in any form or by any means, including photocopying, recording, or other electronic or mechanical methods, without the prior written permission of the publisher, except in the case of brief quotations embodied in critical reviews and certain other noncommercial uses permitted by copyright law.

TABLEOF CONTENTS

INTRODUCTION

CHAPTER 1: UNVEILING THE HISTORY OF WATERCRESS

1.1 Ancient Knowledge, Eternal Cure.

1.2 Watercress in Different Cultures.

1.3 A Sign of Lifeand Renewal.

1.4 Modern Rediscovery and Scientific Validation.

CHAPTER 2: WATERCRESS, A NUTRITIONAL WONDER

2.1 A Rangeof Nutritional Elements.

2.2 Antioxidant Arsenal.

2.3 The Secret Weapon is Glucosinolates.

2.3 Phytonutrients: Mother Nature's Allies.

2.4 Synergy and Wholeness: Beyond the Numbers.

CHAPTER 3: HYDRO-POWER FOR DETOXIFICATION

3.1 The Watercress Cleanse.

3.2 Detoxification and Glucosinolates.

3.3 Cellular Cleansing and Antioxidants.

3.4 Detox and Inflammation Reduction.

3.5 Nourishment from the InsideOut.

CHAPTER 4: WATERCRESS FOR VITALITY AND ENERGY

4.1 The Nutrient Symphony for Energy.

4.2 Iron Vitality and Oxygenation.

4.3 Energy Catalysts are B Vitamins.

4.4 Nutrient Density for Active Lifestyles.

4.5 The Benefits of Watercress for Mental Clarity.

4.6 The Watercress Advantage in SustainableEnergy.

CHAPTER 5: WATERCRESS'S AESTHETIC ADVANTAGES: SKIN, HAIR, AND BEYOND

5.1 TheOuter Reflection of Inner Health.

5.2 Watercress and Skin Health.

5.3 Hair and Nail Nourishment.

5.4 Antioxidants for Gleaming Aging.

5.5 Skin Conditions and Inflammation Reduction.

5.6 Self-Careand Self-Belief: The Watercress Effect.

CHAPTER 6: WATERCRESS COOKING ADVENTURES

6.1 Using Watercress in Regular Meals.

6.2 Colorful Watercress Salads.

6.3 Watercress Soups that areFilling.

6.4 Watercress in Main Dishes.

6.5 Smoothies and Drinks with Watercress.

6.6 Watercress-Infused Drinks:

   6.6.1 Watercress Lemonade.

   6.6.2 Watercress Iced Tea.

   6.6.3 Detox Water with Watercress.

Chapter 7: Practical Incorporation Advice from Science to Plate

- 7.1 Sourcing for Watercress

- 7.2 Proper Storage Procedures

- 7.3 Cleaning and Preparing Watercress

- 7.4 Keeping Flavors Balanced in Recipes

- 7.5 Cooking with Watercress

- 7.6 Meal Preparation and Batch Planning

Chapter 8: Radiate Well-Being with Watercress

- 8.1 A Comprehensive Transformation

- 8.2 Your Personal Watercress Adventure

- 8.3 Taking Careof Your Mind, Body, and Soul

- 8.4 The Persistenceof Radiance

- 8.5 Thankful for the Bounty of Nature

Chapter 9: Navigating Your Watercress Journey

- 9.1 Setting Your Goals for Wellness

- 9.2 Progressive Integration

- 9.3 Supporting Diversity

- 9.4 Consistency is Important

- 9.5 Celebration of Progress

- 9.6 Spreading the Light

- 9.7 Accepting the Road Ahead

Chapter 10: Beyond Words: Your Radiant Future

- 10.1 Write Your Wellness Story

- 10.2 Reimagined Radiance

- 10.3 Wellness Has a RippleEffect

- 10.4 Living in the Hereand Now

- 10.5 Gratitude for Your Radiant Journey

- 10.6 Your Radiance, Your Journey

INTRODUCTION

Utilizing nature's abundance toachieve radiant well-being is more important than ever in a world where wellness is of utmost importance. Welcome to "Revitalize with Watercress: The Ultimate Guide to Radiant Wellness. This thorough guide delves into the nutritional power of watercress and examines how this underappreciated aquatic green may hold the key toa healthier, moreenergetic you. This article seeks to shed light on the potential of watercress to refresh your body, mind, and spirit, from its ancient origins to its contemporary applications.

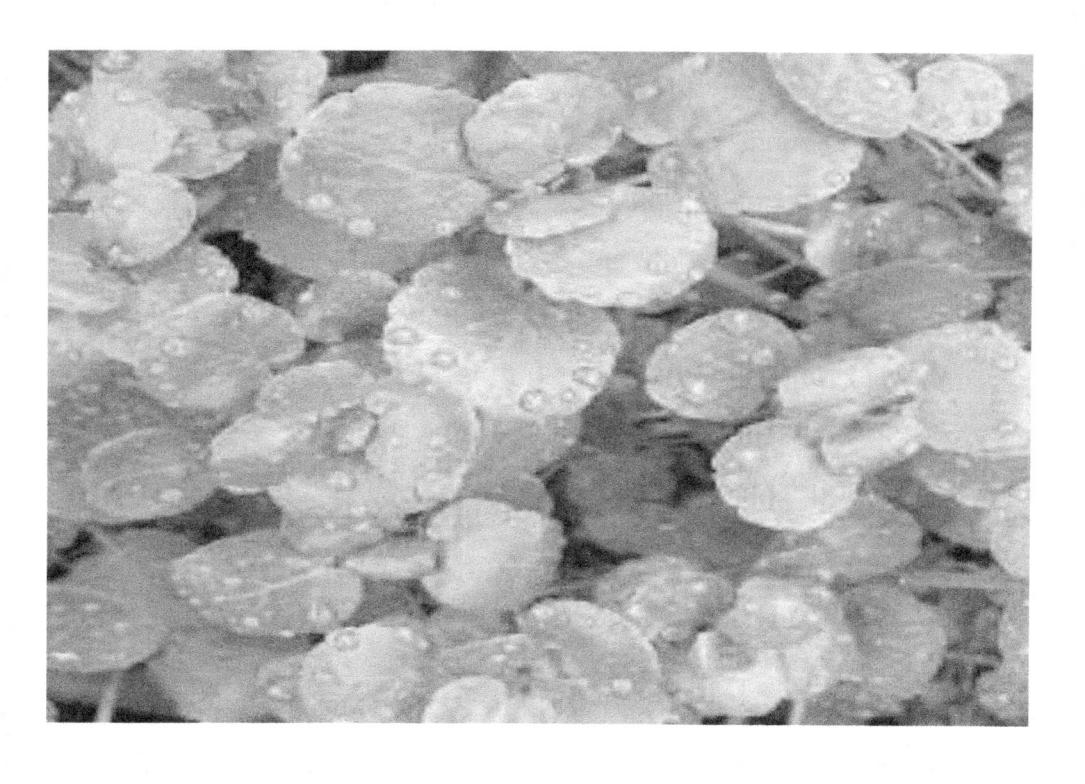

CHAPTER 1

UNVEILING THE HISTORY OF WATERCRESS

The gifts of nature that have sustained humanity for centuries must be reconnected in a world where modern lifestyles frequently push us further away from our origins. Even though it is a common aquatic green, watercress has a long history that crosses all cultures and periods of history. We set out on a journey in this chapter to unravel the historical tapestry that incorporates watercress into the fabric of health and well-being.

Ancient Knowledge, Eternal Cure.

A look at the history of watercress reveals that it was valued by ancient societies long before modern medicine was developed. Watercress was praised for its cleansing abilities and capacity to reestablish balance in the body in traditional healing systems, including Ayurvedaand Traditional Chinese Medicine. We can better understand the reverence with which watercress was regarded as a treatment for various illnesses by understanding its origins in ancient wisdom.

1.2 Watercress in Different Cultures.

Watercress has been embraced by cultures all over the world as a staple food and a healing plant. The versatility of watercress is a testament to its adaptability and cultural significance, from theEuropean tradition of using it in salads and sandwiches to the Japanese practiceof using it in hot pots and soups. We investigate the ways that various cultures have incorporated watercress into their culinary and therapeutic traditions, shedding light on its enduring appeal.

1.3 A sign of lifeand renewal

Due to its preference for wet environments like springs and streams, watercress carries symbolism for *rebirth*and *vitality*. Watercress frequently represented cleansing and rejuvenation in prehistoric mythology and folklore. This chapter explores the myths and symbols associated with watercress, providing insight into theenduring relationships between nature, culture, and well-being.

1.4 Modern Rediscovery and Scientific Validation.

Although the historical importanceof watercress cannot be disputed, current scientific research has opened up a fresh perspectiveon how beneficial it is for our health. The nutritional valueand bioactive substances that contribute to watercress's wellness-improving properties are discussed in this chapter. We come toa comprehensive understanding of the function of watercress in fostering radiant well-being as we bridge the gap between conventional wisdom and empirical support.

The story of watercress is oneof continuity, adaptability, and unfailing capacity to contribute to the welfareof humanity, from ancient healers to contemporary researchers.

CHAPTER 2

WATERCRESS, A NUTRITIONAL WONDER

It's time to delve deeper into the nutritional gold mine that resides within this unassuming aquatic plant. We set out on a journey through the vitamins, minerals, antioxidants, and special compounds in this chapter that make watercress a true superfood and a necessary component on the road to radiant health.

2.1 A Rangeof Nutritional Elements.

Not just any green, watercress is a nutritional powerhouse that is packed with important vitamins and minerals. From calcium to iron, from vitamin A to vitamin K, watercress is a rich sourceof nutrients that support overall health. We'll examine the nutritional profileof watercress and highlight its potential to support a well-rounded diet by completing nutritional gaps.

2.2 Antioxidant Arsenal

The natural defenses against theoxidative stress that our bodies experienceevery day areantioxidants. With its high concentration of antioxidants like vitamin C, beta-carotene, and flavonoids, watercress stands out. These substances combat harmful free radicals, lowering the risk of chronic illnesses and enhancing cellular health. Learn how you can improve your health by utilizing the powerful antioxidant properties of watercress.

2.3 The Secret Weapon is Glucosinolates

Theabundanceof glucosinolates, sulfur-containing compounds that are gaining attention for their potential health benefits, in watercress is among its most intriguing characteristics. Glucosinolates decompose into biologically active compounds with anti-inflammatory and possibly anticancer properties. Examine how glucosinolates support the body's defense mechanisms by learning moreabout the science behind them.

2.3 Phytonutrients: Mother Nature's Allies

The vibrant colors and distinctive flavors of plants area result of phytonutrients, which areorganic substances found in plants. These phytonutrients, which areabundant in watercress and have been linked toa number of health advantages, such as the support of the immune system and anti-inflammatory effects, are very beneficial to human health. Discover how theseorganic allies can help you achieveand sustain radiant health.

2.4 Synergy and Wholeness: Beyond the Numbers

It's important to realize that while individual nutrients and compounds have value, the magic of watercress lies in the interaction of its parts. A holistic nutritional profile that nourishes the body on various levels is produced by the complex interplay of vitamins, minerals, antioxidants, and bioactive substances. You areembracing a wellness symphony when you eat watercress rather than just consuming nutrients.

CHAPTER 3

HYDRO-POWER FOR DETOXIFICATION

The body's natural detoxification processes are more crucial than ever in today's world of environmental toxins and stressors. Theaquatic origins and nutrient-rich makeup of watercress make it an effectiveally in assisting the body's detoxification processes. In this chapter, weexplore the watercress's hydro-powered detoxifying potential and how it can aid in your quest for a vibrant stateof well-being.

3.1 The Watercress Cleanse

Similar to how it aids in internal cleansing, watercress prefers areas with plenty of water. Its high water content hydrates whilealsoacting as a natural diuretic to help the body rid itself of toxins through urination. We look into how watercress's innateability to support the body's natural detoxification processes and maintain healthy kidney function.

3.2 Detoxification and Glucosinolates.

Becauseof its high concentration of glucosinolates, watercress is an effective detoxifier. When these substances are broken down during digestion, they produce isothiocyanates, which have been associated with accelerated liver detoxification procedures. Learn how the body's main detox organ benefits from the glucosinolates in watercress and how they promote general health.

3.3 Cellular Cleansing and Antioxidants.

Detoxification involves more than just getting rid of waste; it also involves defending cells against harm from toxins and free radicals. Vitamins A, C, and E, among other antioxidants in watercress, support the body's defenses against oxidative stress. Learn how theantioxidants in watercress support cellular health and strengthen the body's defenses against toxic assaults.

3.4 Detox and Inflammation Reduction.

Numerous health problems frequently havea chronic inflammatory component. Theanti-inflammatory properties of watercress, which are fueled by ingredients like beta-caroteneand quercetin, areessential for reducing inflammation and easing the strain on the body's detoxification systems. We look at how consuming watercress can foster a peaceful environment that encourages internal wellness.

3.5 Nourishment from the InsideOut.

Providing the body with the nutrients it needs to heal and regenerate is alsoa key component of detoxification. With its nutrient-rich profile, watercress makes sure that your body is not only cleansed but also nourished during the detox process. Learn how this dual-action strategy distinguishes watercress as a natural detoxification aid.

Watercress emerges as a natural ally for how to cleanse, renew, and revitalizeas we navigate the detoxification waters.

CHAPTER 4

WATERCRESS FOR VITALITY AND ENERGY

The pursuit of constant energy and vitality is crucial in our fast-paced lives. With its nutrient-rich makeup and distinctive combination of vitamins and minerals, watercress holds the promiseof energizing your body and mind. This chapter explores how watercress can fuel your daily activities and improve your general wellbeing by acting as a potent sourceof energy.

4.1 The Nutrient Symphony for Energy

The nutrients your body consumes havea complex relationship with vitality. A nutrient symphony that supports efficient energy production is created by theabundanceof vitamins and minerals found in watercress, including B vitamins, iron, and magnesium. Discover how these vital nutrients work together to maintain your energy levels and support metabolic processes.

4.2 Iron Vitality and Oxygenation

A crucial mineral that helps the body transport oxygen is iron. Watercress has a surprising amount of iron, despite looking likea leafy green, which helps the body's cells and tissues absorb oxygen. Learn how the iron in watercress is a hidden gem that can increase your energy and help you fight fatigue.

4.3 Energy catalysts are B vitamins

The B vitamins, also known as theenergy vitamins, are crucial for the body's ability to turn food into fuel. The B vitamin profileof watercress, which includes folateand B6, promotes the metabolism of carbohydrates, proteins, and fats to providea consistent supply of energy. Weexplore how these vitamins function as catalysts for sustaining long-term vitality.

4.4 Nutrient density for active lifestyles

The need for nutrients is greater in people who lead active lifestyles. Athletes and people whoengage in regular physical activity should add watercress to their diets becauseof its exceptional nutrient density. Learn how watercress can support a healthy diet for an active lifestyle whilealso improving performanceand promoting muscle recovery.

4.5 The Benefits of Watercress for Mental Clarity

Being mentally clear is just as important as being physically vibrant. Antioxidants and omega-3 fatty acids found in watercress, as well as other nutrients, support mental health and cognitive function. Learn how watercress can help you focus more clearly, feel better, and have more sustained mental energy.

4.6 The Watercress Advantage in SustainableEnergy

Contrary to caffeine-induced energy spikes, watercress provides steady, balanced energy support. Becauseof its unique nutritional composition, it encourages a steady releaseof energy rather than theabrupt surge that artificial stimulants frequently cause. Learn how adding watercress to your diet can result in all-day energy that lasts.

Additionally, it has come to light that this aquatic green is the key toa balanced and long-lasting sourceof life force.

CHAPTER 5

WATERCRESS'S AESTHETIC ADVANTAGES: SKIN, HAIR, AND BEYOND.

The search for beauty frequently coincides with the pursuit of health. Becauseof its nutrient-rich makeup and special combination of compounds, watercress has benefits for your external appearance in addition to your internal health. This chapter explores how the benefits of watercress extend beyond vitality and help you look radiant, have healthy skin, and have lustrous hair.

5.1 TheOuter Reflection of Inner Health It is undeniable that internal health and outward appearanceare related. Your skin, hair, and nails will be healthier and more vibrant as a result of watercress's high nutritional content. You build a solid foundation for a radiant exterior that reflects your overall vitality by nourishing your body from the insideout.

5.2 Watercress and Skin Health

A canvas for happiness is healthy skin. The high vitamin C, beta-carotene, and antioxidant content of watercress supports overall skin rejuvenation, collagen production, and UV protection, all of which are beneficial for the health of the skin. Learn how watercress can be your ally in achieving a clear, youthful, and glowing complexion.

5.3 Hair and nail nourishment

Strong nails and healthy-looking hair are signs of vitality. The nutritional profileof watercress contains sulfur, silica, and biotin, which are crucial building blocks for healthy hair and nails. Learn how these components help to maintain healthy, strong hair and nails whileavoiding problems like brittleness and hair loss.

5.4 Antioxidants for Gleaming Aging.

Cellular harm and oxidative stress are closely related to theaging process. Antioxidants found in watercress, such as vitamin Eand beta-carotene, serveas a natural deterrent to free radicals, which quicken theaging process. Discover how watercress helps the body fight off early aging and promotes a graceful, youthful appearance.

5.5 Skin Conditions and Inflammation Reduction.

Acne, eczema, and psoriasis area few examples of skin conditions that frequently result from inflammation. By lowering redness, irritation, and flare-ups, watercress's anti-inflammatory properties can bea useful tool in managing these conditions. Find out how the bioactive ingredients in watercress can heal and sooth irritated skin.

5.6 Self-Careand Self-Belief: The Watercress Effect

In addition to improving your physical features, theadvantages of watercress can also improve your emotional and self-esteem by making you look better. It goes hand in hand with feeling good about yourself to feel good about how you look. Discover how incorporating watercress into your self-care routine can improve your stateof mind in general.

It is clear that watercress has many advantages outsideof internal health. The following chapter delves into the fascinating world of culinary explorations with watercress, examining its adaptable use in a variety of dishes that both entice the palateand nourish the body.

CHAPTER 6

WATERCRESS COOKING ADVENTURES

It need not bea chore to includea nutrient-dense food like watercress in your diet; in fact, it can bea delightful culinary adventure. This chapter takes us into the kitchen toexplore some delicious and inventive ways to use watercress in food. Watercress provides a plethoraof culinary and nutritional options, from soups to salads, smoothies to sandwiches.

6.1 Using watercress in regular meals

The peppery and mildly bitter flavor profileof watercress complements a variety of foods. Learn how to incorporate watercress into your regular meals to improve both flavor and nutritional value, whether you'rea seasoned chef or a novice home cook.

6.2 Colorful Watercress Salads.

Watercress gives any salad a zingy, peppery kick and serves as a blank canvas for culinary creativity. Investigate various blendings of ingredients that enhance the flavors, textures, and nutrients of watercress. Find out how to make watercress the star of all your salad creations, from fruity summer salads to hearty grain bowls.

Preparing a watercress salad

Watercress salad is a delicious dish that combines the watercress's peppery, crisp notes with a variety of other fresh ingredients. This salad offers a variety of health advantages in addition to tantalizing the taste buds. Now let's get started on making a tasty and wholesome watercress salad.

Ingredients:

The following is a list of the basic ingredients for a watercress salad.

- 1 bunch of new watercress.
- 1 cup cherry tomatoes.
- 12 cucumbers.
- 14 red onions.
- Optional 1/4 cup of crumbled feta cheese.
- 1/4 cup of toasted nuts, such as almonds or walnuts (optional).

To Dress:

- Two tablespoons of extra-virgin oliveoil.
- 1 tablespoon of lemon juiceor balsamic vinegar.
- One teaspoon of optional Dijon mustard.

- To taste, salt and freshly ground black pepper.

Instructions:

1. Prepare the watercress as follows.

   Start by giving the watercress a thorough rinse under cold running water. Look for and removeany leaves that have yellowed or withered. While young watercress stems are frequently tender enough toeat, you can trim the tough stems if you'd like.

2. Sliceand dice.

   - Sliceeach cherry tomato in half.

   - Cut the cucumber into rounds or half-moons by thinly slicing it.

   - Slice the red onion very thinly. If you find the flavor of raw onion to be too strong, you can mellow it by soaking it in cold water for a short period of time. Before including in the salad, drain.

   - In a dry skillet over medium heat, toast the nuts if you're using them until they're fragrant and just beginning to brown. Consequently, the salad gains a lovely crunch.

3. The salad should be put together as follows.

   - Watercress, cherry tomatoes, cucumber, and red onion should all be combined in a sizable salad bowl. Gently toss them together to combine.

   - If using feta cheeseand toasted nuts, top the salad with them.

4. "Dress It Up".

   - Combine theoliveoil, balsamic vinegar (or lemon juice), and Dijon mustard (if using) ina small bowl. To taste, add salt and pepper to the food. After tasting the dressing, tweak the flavors to your liking.

   - Just before serving, drizzle the dressing over the salad. Be careful not tooverdress; you can always add more if necessary.

   - Gently toss the salad so that the dressing is distributed evenly among the ingredients.

5. Serveand savor:

   Salad should be moved to serving platter or individual plates. To keep the watercress salad fresh and crisp, it is best to serve it right away.

Optional Modifications:

- You can add grilled chicken, shrimp, or tofu for extra protein.

- To createa distinctive textureand flavor, try experimenting with various nuts, such as almonds, walnuts, or pine nuts.

- For a hint of sweetness, add sliced strawberries, orange segments, orapples.

- Add avocado slices for creaminess and good fats.

In addition to being a delicious and energizing dish, watercress salad is a fantastic way to include the health benefits of watercress in your diet. To suit your tasteand dietary needs, feel free to get creative with the ingredients and dressings in your salad. Enjoy your colorful and fresh watercress salad!

6.3 Watercress soups that are filling.

Soups provide comfort and nourishment, and watercress can transform them into nutrient-rich culinary wonders. Learn how to make soups that incorporate the health benefits of this aquatic green, whether it's in the form of a creamy potatoand watercress soup or a reviving green detox soup.

Preparation of watercress Soup

A warm bowl of soup and the distinctively peppery flavor of watercress are combined in watercress soup, a dish that is light and refreshing. In addition to being delicious, it is alsoa great sourceof vitamins and minerals. Let's look at how to make this flavorful and nourishing soup.

Ingredients:

You'll need the following ingredients to makea simple watercress soup:.

– One bunch of fresh watercress.

- 1 medium-sized potato, diced after being peeled.

- a chopped one-small onion.

- Two minced cloves of garlic.

– 4 cups of vegetableor chicken broth.

- 2 tablespoons of oliveoil or butter.

- As needed, freshly ground black pepper and salt.

- An optional garnish of a little cream or yogurt.

Instructions:

1. Prepare the watercress as follows.

- To begin, give the watercress a good rinse under cold running water. Eliminateany wilted, yellowed, or tough stems. The tender stems can be left on since cooking will make them softer.

2. Aromatics should be sautéed.

- Melt the butter or oliveoil in a large soup pot over medium heat. Add the minced garlic and onion, both chopped.

Theonion and garlic should be sautéed for about 2-3 minutes, or until they are translucent and fragrant.

3. Potato is added.

- Add the diced potato to the pot and cook for an additional two to three minutes while stirring.

4. Simmer while using broth.

- Cover the potatoes completely with the vegetableor chicken broth. If necessary, add a little water to make sure the potatoes are completely submerged.

- Heat the mixture until it boils, then lower the heat so that it simmers. For about 15-20 minutes, or until the potatoes areeasily pierced with a fork, simmer the mixture with the lid on.

5. Use the watercress in your dish.

- After the potatoes are finished cooking, add the watercress that has been rinsed to the pot.

- Stir well, allowing the watercress to wilt and combine with theother ingredients.

6. Smoothly blend.

- Carefully blend the soup using an immersion blender or a standard blender (in batches) until it is smooth and creamy. When blending soup in a regular blender, be sure to let the soup cool slightly first.

- Toachieve the desired consistency, add a little bit more broth or water if the soup is too thick.

7. Add seasoning and garnish.

- Taste the soup and adjust the seasoning as desired with salt and freshly ground black pepper.

- Toadd more creaminess, if desired, whisk in a splash of cream or yogurt.

8. Serving and enjoying:

Pour the watercress soup into bowls and add a few fresh watercress leaves for a more posh finishing touch. Serve this nourishing soup hot and enjoy the wonderful flavor combination and nutritional value.

Alternatives include:

- Add a squeezeof lemon juice right before serving for a zesty and vibrant twist.

- Experiment with various herbs and spices to improve the flavor profile, such as thyme, tarragon, or nutmeg.

- You can add cooked rice, quinoa, or lentils to make the soup heartier.

It is possible to customize watercress soup to your personal tastes because it is a flexible dish. It'sa great way to incorporate the distinctive qualities of watercress into your culinary repertoire while savoring its delicious flavor and health advantages, whether eaten as an appetizer or a light main course.

6.4 Watercress in Main Dishes.

Watercress can take the lead in your main courses rather than just serving as a garnish. Learn how to include watercress as a featured ingredient in stir-fries, pasta dishes, andother dishes to give your favorite foods a burst of flavor and nutrition.

6.5 Smoothies and Drinks with Watercress

Watercress can also beadded to your favorite drinks if you prefer to sip your nutrients. Discover smoothie recipes that incorporate watercress along with other superfoods, fruits, and vegetables to create scrumptious concoctions that nourish your body from the insideout.

Making drinks and smoothies with watercress.

Watercress can infuse your beverages with flavor and nutrients, so it's not just for salads. We'll look at how to make hydrating smoothies and drinks that highlight the flavorful qualities and health advantages of watercress in this guide.

Ingredients for a basic watercress smoothie:

- 1 cup of fresh watercress, including the stems and leaves.

- 1 ripe banana.

- A dairy-free yogurt substituteor 1/2 cup of Greek yogurt.

- 1/2 cup of the milk of your choice (dairy, almond, soy, etc.).

- 1 tablespoon of maple syrup or honey (optional for sweetness).

- Ice cubes, optionally added for thickness.

Instructions:

1. Prepare the watercress as follows:

- Start by giving the watercress a thorough rinse under cold running water. Removeany wilted or yellowed leaves as well as the stronger stems. Stems that are tender and blend well can beadded.

2. Mix the ingredients.

- Blend together the fresh watercress, ripe banana, milk, Greek yogurt (or a dairy-free substitute), and sweetener (if desired).

If you want your smoothie to be thicker and colder, add a few ice cubes.

3. Until smooth, blend:

- Blend all of the ingredients until a smooth, creamy mixture results. This may require 1-2 minutes depending on your blender.

4. Contextualize sweetness and consistency.

- You can adjust the consistency of your smoothie by adding more milk if it is too thick.

- Taste the smoothieand, if you'd like it sweeter, add more honey or maple syrup.

5. "Serveand Enjoy.".

Serve the watercress smoothie right away after pouring it intoa glass. For a classy finishing touch, garnish with a fresh watercress sprig.

Alternatives include:

- For a fruity twist, add a few handfuls of berries (such as strawberries, blueberries, or raspberries).

- Includea tablespoon of chiaor flaxseeds for more fiber and omega-3 fatty acids.

- For a zesty kick, add a squeezeof limeor lemon juice to the dish toenhance the flavor.

6.6 Watercress-Infused Drinks:

Watercress can also be incorporated into various drinks:

1. *"Watercress Lemonade".*

Watercress-infused lemonade can be made by blending fresh watercress with lemon juice, water, and sweetener. Before serving, strain.

2. *"Watercress Iced Tea".*

- Let watercress leaves steep in hot water for a few minutes before cooling. Squeezea little lemon juiceand sweetener in for flavor.

3. *Detox Water with Watercress:*

- In a pitcher of water, mix watercress leaves, cucumber slices, lemon wedges, and mint leaves. For a detoxifying beverage, let the flavors steep overnight.

Play around with different combinations and flavors to make smoothies and drinks that suit your palate while taking advantageof the many health advantages that watercress offers your sips. Cheers to reviving your drinks with watercress's peppery goodness!

CHAPTER 7

PRACTICAL INCORPORATION ADVICE FROM SCIENCE TO PLATE

Given the impressive health advantages and culinary versatility of watercress, it's time to put theory into practice. This chapter offers you helpful suggestions on how to incorporate watercress into your daily routine. These suggestions will help you get the most out of this nutrient-rich aquatic gem, from choosing the freshest bunches to cooking delectable meals.

7.1 Sourcing for watercress.

Choosing premium watercress is the first step on the path to culinary and health success. Recognize fresh bunches by their vibrant leaves and stems. We investigate the best watercress sources, from farmers' markets to supermarkets, to make sure you get off toa good watercress start.

7.2 Proper Storage Procedures

Proper storage is necessary to protect the nutritional integrity of watercress. Learn how to keep it crisp and flavorful for as long as possibleand increase the shelf lifeof your food. Weoffer suggestions for keeping your watercress fresh, such as putting it in the refrigerator or placing a glass of water on the counter.

7.3 Cleaning and preparing watercress

Cleaning watercress thoroughly to get rid of any contaminants or dirt is essential before utilizing its health benefits. Washing and preparing watercress for use in salads, soups, and other dishes requires careful attention to detail. Wealso talk about the stems, which have some nutritional valueof their own and have some creative uses.

7.4 Keeping Flavors Balanced in Recipes

The distinct peppery flavor of watercress can bea wonderful addition to your dishes, but it's important to balance its flavor with other ingredients. Learn how to incorporatewatercress into dishes with complementary flavors, textures, and seasonings to makeeach onea delicious symphony of tasteand nutrition.

7.5 Cooking with Watercress

Watercress can producea variety of textures and flavors by using various cooking techniques. Learn how to maximize the culinary potential of watercress by using methods like quick sautés and gentle wilting. For recipes that taste great and are nutritious, wealsooffer adviceon when toadd watercress.

7.6 Meal preparation and batch planning

With careful meal planning and batch cooking, incorporating watercress into your routine becomes simple. Learn how to incorporate watercress into your weekly menu in order to save timeand ensure that you regularly benefit from it. Wealsooffer adviceon how to prepare meals for busy days with watercress.

CHAPTER 8

RADIATE WELL-BEING WITH WATERCRESS

It's time to consider how this aquatic treasure has affected every aspect of your health. The highlights of our investigation are reviewed in this last chapter, and we offer some final suggestions on how you can embrace radiant health by incorporating watercress into your daily routine.

8.1 A Comprehensive Transformation.

Watercress has repeatedly shown its capacity to improve wellbeing on a variety of levels, as evidenced by both historical practices and contemporary scientific validation. Recall the most important lessons learned from each chapter, including its history, culinary diversity, and the many ways it can support your health and vitality.

8.2 Your Personal Watercress Adventure

Your experience with watercress is special and individual to you. Watercress can be your trustworthy companion whether you're looking for detoxification, vitality, enhanced appearance, or all of the above. Consider your personal objectives and how watercress relates to your desire for wellness, realizing that it has the power to improve your journey.

8.3: Taking careof your mind, body, and soul

The health advantages of watercress extend past the physical realm and alsoaffect your mental and emotional well-being. Adopt the perspective that you arealso nourishing your mind and soul as you provide your body with the nutrients it needs. This all-encompassing method of well-being lays the groundwork for a life that is more symmetrical and harmonious.

8.4 The Persistenceof Radiance

Keep in mind that achieving radiant health requires continued effort as you incorporate watercress into your daily routine. Your wellbeing increases when you consistently give your body the nutrients it needs, just as watercress does in its aquatic habitat. Accept watercress as a sign of rebirth and a constant reminder to put your health first.

8.5 Thankful for the bounty of nature

The journey that watercress takes from the stream to the plate is evidenceof nature's wonders. Thank it for the nourishment it brings, for the knowledge of the past, and for the understanding of the present. Realize how deeply you are a part of nature and how marvelously it helps you on your path to radiance.

CHAPTER 9

NAVIGATING YOUR WATERCRESS JOURNEY

It's crucial to have a road map for exploring and incorporating this aquatic treasure into your life. We give you helpful advice and pointers in this chapter to help you manage your ongoing relationship with watercress and make sure its advantages continue to improve your well-being.

9.1 Setting Your Goals for Wellness

Setting specific intentions for your wellbeing at the outset of your watercress journey will help. Determining your objectives gives you a sense of purpose that motivates you to incorporate watercress into your lifestyle, whether you're aiming for better vitality, clearer skin, or increased energy levels.

9.2 Progressive Integration

A sustainable wellness regimen cannot be created overnight, just as Rome was not. As you begin to incorporate watercress into your diet, try out various preparations and recipes. As you gradually enjoy its advantages, this strategy enables you to train your palate to its distinctive flavors and textures.

9.3 Supporting Diversity.

Theendless culinary possibilities made possible by watercress's adaptability. Rotate watercress into various dishes and meals toembrace variety. By doing this, you can avoid becoming monotonous and guarantee that you consumea variety of flavors and nutrients.

9.4 Consistency is Important.

Any successful wellness initiative must be based on consistency. Attempt to include watercress frequently in your diet. This could entail planning meals with watercress as the main ingredient, keeping watercress on hand for quick use, or just developing a habit of mindful eating.

9.5 Celebration of progress.

Takea moment toacknowledge your accomplishments as you begin to feel the benefits of watercress on your health. Recognizing theadvantages, whether they be increased energy, clearer skin, or a renewed senseof vitality, strengthens your resolve to continueon the path.

The watercress journey is a never-ending path of exploration; it doesn't end with this guide. Continue discovering new uses for watercress, experimenting with new dishes, and remaining receptive to its ever-evolving advantages. Keep learning moreabout its nutritional valueand potential uses.

9.6 Spreading the Light.

Consider telling your friends, family, and other loved ones about your watercress journey as you succeed. Your enthusiasm may spur others to start their own wellness journeys, resulting in a chain reaction of wellness and vitality.

9.7 Accepting the Road Ahead.

Keep in mind that the watercress journey you'reon is a dynamic, ever-changing process as you travel it. Seize theopportunities this journey presents to learn, to taste, and to discover. In theend, the road to radiant health is paved by your deliberateactions and the nourishing gifts of nature.

CHAPTER 10

BEYOND WORDS: YOUR RADIANT FUTURE

In closing, keep in mind that this is only the beginning of a radiant and transformative journey with "The Ultimate Guide to Radiant Well-being." Your future will beone that glistens with happiness, vitality, and brilliance, and the words on these pages aremerely signposts directing you in that direction. This chapter's invitation encourages you to think beyond the text and consider your own untapped potential.

10.1 Write Your Wellness Story

You are theauthor of your wellness memoir, and watercress is a key element. Every meal, bite, and decision you makeas time goes on will eventually paint a different color on the canvas of your health. Accept this journey as an ongoing story that changes as you continue to discover, gain knowledge, and develop.

10.2 Reimagined Radiance

Imagine waking up every day with a renewed senseof vitality, a clear mind, and a body that feels aliveand energized. Try to picture your skin glowing with happiness when you look in the mirror. Imagine yourself meeting life's challenges with fortitude, resiliency, and a clear head, all propelled by the sustaining power of watercress.

10.3 Wellness Has a RippleEffect

Your light radiates out toaffect the lives of those close to you as you live by the principles of well-being. Your improved health may motivate loved ones, friends, and coworkers to start their own journeys to wellness. Your useof watercress benefits both your personal health and the health of your community in this way.

10.4 Living in the Hereand Now.

Always keep in mind that happiness is a continuous journey that takes place in each moment. Embrace the moment, whether you'reenjoying a salad with watercress, engaging in mindfulness, or taking careof yourself. You have the chance to feed your body, mind, and soul in every moment.

10.5 Gratitude for Your Radiant Journey

Thank God for the knowledge gained, the discoveries made, and the transformation that lies ahead as you close this book. Beappreciativeof tradition's wisdom, the thrill of self-discovery, and the guidance provided by watercress. Your journey is infused with gratitude, which also creates the foundation for long-term well-being.

10.6 Your Radiance, Your Journey

In theend, you are theone who defines and explores the path to radiant well-being. The foundation has been laid by "Revitalize with Watercress: The Ultimate Guide to Radiant Well-Being," but your journey is entirely your own. The sameenthusiasm and curiosity with which you haveembraced watercress, embraceeach chapter of your life. Let your journey serveas an exampleof how mindful living, conscious decision-making, and the close relationship between natureand well-being can all have transformativeeffects.